COMPLETE GUIDE TO GANGLION CYST REMOVAL

Comprehensive Handbook To Expert Techniques, Home Remedies, And Post Surgery Care For Pain Relief And Healing

DR. BRUNO HORAN

Disclaimer:

The information provided in this book, is intended for general informational purposes only and should not be considered as professional advice.

The author has made every effort to ensure the accuracy of the information presented. However, readers are advised to consult with a qualified healthcare professional before attempting any herbal remedies or making significant changes to their wellness routine. Individual health conditions vary, and what may be suitable for one person may not be appropriate for another.

It is important to note that the author is not in any endorsement deal, partnership, or affiliation with any organization, brand, or company mentioned in this book. Any references to specific products or services are based on the author's personal experience or general knowledge and do not imply an endorsement or promotion of those products or services

Contents

CONCERNING THIS BOOK

"Ganglion Cyst Removal" is a book that is a valuable resource for individuals and medical professionals who are dealing with this prevalent yet sometimes misdiagnosed illness. Ganglion cysts are fluid-filled sacs that are usually seen near tendons and joints. They can be uncomfortable and interfere with day-to-day activities. It is essential to comprehend their nature, and this book does a fantastic job of demystifying every facet, from identification to treatment.

The book starts by thoroughly defining ganglion cysts and then explores their causes as well as the warning indicators that should prompt a visit to the doctor. The focus is on early detection, highlighting how crucial prompt intervention is to avert consequences. The thorough summary of available treatments, which range from non-surgical methods like aspiration and observation to surgical methods like arthroscopic and open procedures, clarifies the appropriate course of action based on the characteristics and location of the cyst.

Understanding anatomy is essential to comprehending how ganglion cysts develop and affect joint function. Thorough descriptions clarify the many kinds of cysts and how they affect the tissues around them, giving readers vital information for both diagnostic and therapy selection. The process of diagnosis is thoroughly examined, emphasizing the importance of medical history, imaging modalities such as MRI and ultrasound, and physical examinations in accurately identifying the presence of cysts.

The book provides thoughtful talks on methods like immobilization and medication, weighing advantages and disadvantages, for individuals considering non-surgical options. Surgical options are equally comprehensive, emphasizing risks, procedural variations, indications, and techniques for post-operative care. The story is further enhanced with case studies and patient testimonies, which provide firsthand accounts of treatment results and recovery processes.

The book answers commonly asked questions about recurrence, recovery timelines, prevention measures, and alternative therapies clearly and compassionately throughout its pages. The impact of ganglion cysts on day-to-day functioning is poignantly brought to light by patient experiences, underscoring the significance of comprehensive care and available resources.

To sum up, "Ganglion Cyst Removal" serves as a clinical guidebook as well as a source of knowledge and direction for everybody who is impacted by these cysts. It improves the conversation about this illness by offering a comprehensive perspective that combines medical knowledge with sympathetic patient-centered viewpoints. This book is not only educational; it is transforming, giving readers the tools they need to confidently and navigate the difficult world of managing ganglion cysts.

The structure and operation of ganglion cells

Non-cancerous tumors called ganglion cysts usually develop along the tendons or joints of the hands or wrists, though they can also develop in other regions of the body. An understanding of the anatomy of tendons and joints is essential to comprehending the development of these cysts. The junction of two or more bones is called a joint, which permits flexibility and movement. Tendons, which are strong bands of tissue that attach muscles to bones, encircle these joints.

The tissues of a joint or tendon may become irritated or inflamed when there is stress or damage, such as from repetitive motions or injury. This inflammation may cause a ganglion cyst to develop. A ganglion cyst is essentially a sac that emerges from the tendon sheath or joint capsule and is filled with a viscous, jelly-like substance. This fluid resembles the synovial fluid that coats and lubricates tendons and joints.

The Reason Behind Cyst Formation in Tendons and Joints

Although the precise etiology of ganglion cyst formation is unknown, it is thought to arise from the deterioration or degeneration of the tissues around tendons or joints.

Wear and strain over time, injuries, or even repetitive stress can cause this collapse. The synovial fluid seeps out of the joint capsule or tendon sheath and produces a cystic formation. In essence, a ganglion cyst is the body attempting self-healing, albeit in an unusual and perhaps difficult method.

Different Ganglion Cyst Types Depending on Location

Although ganglion cysts can develop anywhere, they are most frequently found close to tendons and joints that are stressed or subjected to repetitive activity. The most common locations are the fingers, foot, and wrist, especially on the back of the hand. These cysts typically develop on the dorsal (back) side of the wrist, although they can also occur on the palmar (palm) side or even inside the joint.

Apart from the hand and wrist, ganglion cysts can also form near other joints including the ankle, knee, shoulder, or even along the spine. Usually, their placement is about regions of high mechanical stress and movement.

The Impact of Cysts on Joint Function

The joint function may be impacted by ganglion cysts in several ways. First of all, the cyst itself could hurt or create discomfort, particularly if it presses against surrounding nerves or restricts the range of motion of tendons. Sometimes the cyst might generate a noticeable bulge that affects the appearance of the affected area, or it can impair joint motion.

In terms of functionality, a ganglion cyst can limit movement by producing a mechanical impediment or by producing discomfort during specific activities. For example, a cyst around the wrist joint may cause pain or difficulty when the hand is bent backward (dorsiflexion) or when weight is applied to the wrist. In a similar vein, a cyst close to a finger joint may make it difficult to fully bend or grip the finger.

Typical Areas Where Ganglion Cysts Occur

The hands and wrists are most frequently affected by ganglion cysts, especially the dorsal side of the wrist. They may also show up on the fingers, particularly in the joints that are closest to the nail beds. Apart from these regions, ganglion cysts can also develop on the feet, especially on the ball of the foot or in the vicinity of the ankle joint.

The frequent movements and mechanical strain that these joints and tendons experience during daily activities are mostly to blame for the high incidence of ganglion cysts in these regions.

Cysts, however, may develop in any joint or tendon sheath in the body that experiences comparable trauma or stress.

Effect on Adjacent Tissues

There are various ways that a ganglion cyst might affect the tissues around it. Initially, the cyst may compress adjacent anatomical systems like blood vessels or nerves, resulting in discomfort, tingling, or numbness in the impacted region.

Additionally, the function of tendons may be impacted by this compression, which may impede their capacity to move freely inside their sheaths and result in pain or stiffness.

Furthermore, ganglion cyst pressure on nearby tissues can cause inflammatory reactions, which exacerbates symptoms even more. In certain instances, the cyst could enlarge to the point where it obstructs normal joint function or changes the form of the affected area.

While controlling ganglion cysts primarily aims to relieve pressure on surrounding tissues and restore normal joint function, it is important to be aware of these potential effects when weighing treatment options.

CHAPTER ONE

GANGLION CYST DIAGNOSIS

Clinical Evaluation And Physical Examination

First, a medical practitioner must perform a comprehensive physical examination to diagnose a ganglion cyst. The doctor will closely examine the lump during this examination, noting its size, shape, and placement. A pea to a golf ball in size, ganglion cysts are usually spherical or oval. To determine the cyst's firmness and mobility, the doctor will also feel it. Because ganglion cysts frequently involve joints or tendons, moving the afflicted joint may be part of the evaluation to see if there is any pain or restriction in movement.

As ganglion cysts are known to be filled with fluid, palpation—or gently pressing on the cyst—helps ascertain whether it is. A transillumination test, in which light is flashed through the cyst, may also be performed by the physician. The diagnosis of a ganglion cyst is supported if the light penetrates and lights the cyst, indicating that the cyst is filled with fluid.

Imaging Methodologies For Precise Diagnosis

Even while a physical examination can offer important hints, imaging methods are frequently used to get a more precise diagnosis.

An ultrasound is a non-invasive imaging method that makes images of internal body structures by using sound waves. It is especially helpful in separating fluid-filled cysts from solid objects and verifying their existence.

Assessing the cyst's connection to other tissues, such as tendons and joints, can also be done with ultrasound.

Another imaging technique that offers fine-grained pictures of soft tissues is magnetic resonance imaging

(MRI). When the diagnosis is unclear or the cyst is deeply embedded, MRI is quite helpful. It can show the precise position, size, and form of the cyst as well as how it is connected to neighboring structures. Additionally useful in ruling out other possible diagnoses, MRI can be used to rule out soft tissue anomalies or malignancies.

Differential Diagnosis Using Additional Masses And Lumps

It is essential to distinguish ganglion cysts from other kinds of lumps and masses to administer treatment appropriately. Although sebaceous cysts, lipomas (fatty tumors), and even malignant tumors can manifest as bumps, ganglion cysts are benign and fluid-filled masses. The medical professional will consider these options while diagnosing.

For example, ganglion cysts are typically more mobile and harder than lipomas. Conversely, sebaceous cysts frequently contain a cheesy material within and may have a punctum, or small aperture, on the surface. In addition to being more hard and asymmetrical in shape, malignant tumors can also cause other systemic symptoms including weight loss or nocturnal sweats. The physical features help the practitioner differentiate ganglion cysts from various other illnesses in addition to imaging results.

Medical History Is Important For Diagnosis

A thorough medical history is essential for the diagnosis of ganglion cysts. The length of the lump, any size changes, and any accompanying symptoms like pain or tingling will all be questioned by the medical professional.

Inquiries on past injuries and repetitive activities in the afflicted area will also be made, as these factors have been linked to the development of ganglion cysts.

The doctor will also go over any previous illnesses, prescriptions, and family history of lumps or cysts of a similar nature. This information gives context for the imaging and physical findings and aids in ruling out other illnesses. The diagnosis of a ganglion cyst might be supported by patterns or risk factors found in a comprehensive medical history.

Aspiration's Function In Verifying The Presence Of Cysts

Aspiration is a diagnostic process in which fluid from the cyst is removed with a needle. In addition to relieving symptoms, this treatment confirms the existence of a ganglion cyst.

The medical professional removes the cyst's fluid by carefully threading a thin needle into it while maintaining sterility. Usually transparent and jelly-like, the fluid is indicative of a ganglion cyst.

In addition to confirming the diagnosis, aspiration might temporarily lower the cyst's size, reducing pressure and discomfort. It's crucial to remember, though, that cysts frequently reappear following aspiration. To rule out infection or other diseases, the fluid may be sent to a laboratory for additional investigation if it is not clear or has an unusual appearance. Aspiration is a simple process that aids in the planning of additional care and offers instant insights into the nature of the mass.

CHAPTER TWO

OTHER TRADITIONAL MEDICINE

Asymptomatic Cysts: Monitoring And Observation

Observing and monitoring a tiny ganglion cyst that is not causing discomfort or interfering with normal activities is a popular method.

The doctor will examine the cyst at routine check-ups to look for any changes in size or symptoms. This approach is advantageous since it prevents needless procedures, particularly in cases where the cyst is asymptomatic and does not limit movement.

Patients are urged to report any new symptoms that may require a different course of treatment, such as increased size, pain, or trouble moving a joint.

Methods Of Immobilization To Decrease Cyst Size

An efficient non-surgical treatment for ganglion cyst discomfort in patients is immobilization. The affected area is maintained stationary by wearing a brace or splint, which minimizes movement that can aggravate the cyst.

 By lowering the cyst's internal fluid production, this technique can gradually help shrink the cyst. Because wrist cysts can worsen with repeated motion, immobilization is very helpful in treating these conditions. To prevent joint stiffness or muscle weakening, a healthcare provider should oversee the long-term usage of immobilization devices.

Utilizing Anti-Inflammatories As Medicines To Reduce Pain

Over-the-counter analgesics like ibuprofen or naproxen are commonly used to treat the pain and inflammation brought on by ganglion cysts. By easing pain and reducing swelling, these drugs improve the comfort of daily tasks. When over-the-counter remedies are insufficient, physicians may in some situations recommend stronger anti-inflammatory medications.

Patients should carefully follow dosage guidelines and talk to their healthcare provider about any concerns they may have, especially if they are taking other medications or have other medical issues.

Methods Of Aspiration Used To Remove Cyst Fluid

Aspiration offers instant relief from symptoms like pressure and discomfort by using a needle to remove fluid from the ganglion cyst.

This is a rather simple operation that is usually done in a doctor's office. To reduce discomfort, a local anesthetic is used to numb the area surrounding the cyst. Aspiration is a useful method for symptom relief and a large reduction in cyst size; nevertheless, it is crucial to remember that cysts might return after aspiration. If the cyst recurs, more treatment options may need to be explored. Multiple aspirations may be necessary.

Advantages And Drawbacks Of Non-Surgical Methods

There are various advantages to non-surgical ganglion cyst treatments. They carry fewer dangers, are less invasive than surgical treatments, and typically need a shorter recovery period.

For many patients, these non-surgical treatments can effectively manage symptoms and enhance quality of life. Non-surgical techniques do, however, have certain drawbacks.

They might not offer a long-term fix because cysts might return following procedures like aspiration. Furthermore, some cysts may still cause pain or functional damage even when non-surgical treatments don't work properly.

Surgery might be suggested in some situations to offer a more conclusive outcome.

Comprehending the diverse non-invasive therapeutic alternatives for ganglion cysts enables patients and medical professionals to make knowledgeable choices regarding the most suitable management approaches, taking into account unique situations and inclinations.

CHAPTER THREE

SURGICAL CHORES FOR REMOVAL OF GANGLION CYST

Surgical Intervention Indications

Non-cancerous lumps called ganglion cysts usually form on the tendons or joints of the hands or wrists, although they can also form on the ankles or feet. Although many ganglion cysts dissolve on their own and can be treated conservatively, in some cases surgery is required.

Surgery may be necessary if there is ongoing pain, limited joint mobility, severe discomfort, or when the cyst interferes with day-to-day functioning.

In addition, surgery might be suggested to relieve the cyst and stop further consequences if it keeps coming back despite previous therapies such as aspiration, or if the diagnosis is unclear.

Distinctive Methods of Surgery (Open versus Arthroscopic)

There are two main methods for surgically removing a ganglion cyst: open surgery and arthroscopic surgery.

Open Surgery: In this conventional technique, the cyst is cut open straight across its surface. To reduce the likelihood of a recurrence, the surgeon can then access the entire cyst and remove it, including its stalk or root.

Accurate removal of the cyst may be possible with open surgery since it offers a clear view of the cyst and its surrounding components.

However, compared to less invasive methods, it usually requires a wider incision and could require a longer recovery period.

Arthroscopic Surgery: This minimally invasive procedure entails creating smaller incisions for the insertion of specialized equipment and a tiny camera, known as an arthroscope. Using a monitor to observe the inside of the joint, the surgeon carefully eliminates the cyst.

Smaller scars, a quicker recovery, and less pain following surgery are common outcomes of arthroscopic surgery.

However, not all ganglion cysts are suitable for this procedure, and it requires specialist knowledge and tools.

The Dangers And Issues Related To Surgery

Ganglion cyst removal has several risks and potential problems, just like any surgical surgery. Bleeding, anesthesia-related adverse reactions, and surgical site infection are common hazards.

Damage to the nerves or blood vessels may also occur, which could result in numbness, tingling, or weakening in the affected area. More worries include stiffness and scar development.

The most prominent side effect associated with ganglion cyst surgery is the possibility of the cyst returning, even in cases where the treatment is carried out appropriately.

Patients should evaluate these risks against the benefits of the treatment and discuss them with their surgeon.

After-Operative Treatment And Recovery

For patients to heal well after having a ganglion cyst removed, proper post-operative care is essential. Patients may initially have some discomfort and swelling, but these can be controlled with ice packs and painkillers as directed.

To avoid infection, the surgical site must be kept dry and clean. It might be advised to wear a brace or splint to immobilize the joint and aid in recovery.

To assist regain strength, flexibility, and range of motion, physical therapy frequently plays a vital part in rehabilitation.

Exercises designed specifically for the affected joint can guarantee a return to normal function and prevent stiffness.

It's crucial to schedule routine follow-up visits with the surgeon to track recovery and quickly treat any issues.

Anticipated Results And Recuperation Schedule

The length of recovery following ganglion cyst excision varies based on the surgical approach taken and the health of the patient.

After arthroscopic surgery, patients can usually return to mild activities in a few days to a week, whereas open surgery may need a longer initial recovery period.

In a few weeks to a few months, the majority of patients can resume their regular activities, including work and leisure. To guarantee the best possible recovery, it's critical to follow the post-operative instructions and show up for all follow-up appointments.

Although most patients report significant symptom relief and better joint function, recurrence of the cyst is a possibility and should be discussed with the surgeon.

CHAPTER FOUR

REMOVAL OF ARTHROSCOPIC GANGLION CYST

Comprehensive Arthroscopic Surgery Process

A minimally invasive surgical technique called arthroscopic ganglion cystectomy is used to treat ganglion cysts that form around tendons or joints. The patient is put under anesthesia at the start of the surgery to ensure their comfort.

To insert an arthroscope—a thin tube with a camera and light source—a small incision is made close to the cyst. This enables the surgeon to see the cyst and the surrounding structures in real-time on a monitor.

The surgeon removes the ganglion cyst gently by making additional small incisions and inserting specialized equipment.

Arthroscopy has the advantage of being precise and causing the least amount of tissue disruption possible. By lowering the possibility of harm to surrounding blood vessels and nerves, this technique expedites healing and recovery.

After the cyst is removed, adhesive strips or sutures are usually used to seal the incisions. In many situations, the entire surgery is done as an outpatient, meaning that patients can go home the same day with little to no discomfort.

Benefits Of Less Invasive Techniques

Comparing minimally invasive methods with open surgery, such as arthroscopy, has several benefits. First of all, they require fewer incisions, which lessens scarring and pain following surgery. These methods also lessen the possibility of infection and other problems brought on by bigger incisions. Compared to standard surgery, patients frequently recover more quickly and can return to their regular activities sooner.

Arthroscopy's finely detailed imaging guarantees that surgeons can precisely target the cyst while protecting the surrounding healthy tissue. This accuracy is especially important in sensitive locations like joints, where preserving joint function is critical to the success of the treatment.

Furthermore, increased postoperative mobility and function are a result of minimally invasive techniques' decreased damage to muscles and ligaments. Due to fewer problems and an overall smoother healing period, patients usually report higher levels of satisfaction.

Tools And Equipment Used In Surgery

It needs specialist equipment designed for minimally invasive treatments to remove an arthroscopic ganglion cyst. One of the most important tools is the arthroscope, which has a light source and a camera inside to show the surgery site clearly. Through a tiny incision, the surgeon inserts this device, which gives them precise control over tool navigation and manipulation.

Additional devices utilized in the process include tiny surgical tools made for handling fragile tissue and removing cysts. Further tiny incisions are made surrounding the cyst site to accommodate the insertion of these tools. With the least amount of damage to the surrounding tissues, the surgeon can precisely find and remove the cyst thanks to advanced imaging technologies.

Throughout the surgery, the surgical team makes use of sterile drapes, irrigation systems, and specialized monitors to preserve a clear field of view and track the patient's vital signs. With the use of these instruments, ganglion cysts can be safely and successfully removed using minimally invasive techniques.

Recuperation Procedure After Arthroscopic Excision

After arthroscopic excision of ganglion cysts, patients usually have a simple recuperation period. Patients are kept under observation in a recovery area until they are stable and completely awake following surgery. Medication is one type of pain management strategy that can help during the early stages of recovery.

To enhance joint mobility and prevent stiffness, patients are typically urged to start physical therapy exercises and mild movement at an early age. To minimize the need for follow-up wound care, the small incisions are usually closed with adhesive strips or dissolvable sutures.

A few days to a week following surgery, depending on their particular healing rates and the location of the cyst, is when most patients can resume light activities. It can take several weeks to fully recuperate, including getting back to more physically demanding activities. Scheduling routine check-ups with the surgeon guarantees that the healing process is proceeding according to plan.

Success Rates And Case Studies

The effectiveness and positive results of arthroscopic ganglion cyst excision are demonstrated by case studies and success rates.

According to studies, cyst removal has a high success rate and a low recurrence rate. Following surgery, patients frequently report great alleviation from symptoms like pain and stiffness around the afflicted joint.

The increased popularity of arthroscopy among surgeons and patients alike can be attributed to its ability to accurately target and remove cysts while preserving joint function.

Overall, results are consistently positive, while success rates vary based on factors such as cyst size, location, and unique patient characteristics.

Comparing arthroscopic ganglion cyst removal to open surgery techniques, the former has shown reduced complication rates in clinical settings.

The smaller incisions and less damage to the surrounding tissues are primarily responsible for this. Case studies support the procedure's effectiveness in enhancing patients' quality of life by successfully regaining joint function and reducing symptoms.

CHAPTER FIVE

GANGLION CYST REMOVAL BY OPEN SURGERY

An Overview Of Conventional Open Surgery

An established method for removing ganglion cysts is open surgery, which is employed when the cyst is big, complicated, or situated in a hard-to-reach place where arthroscopic methods would not be appropriate.

In contrast to arthroscopy, which uses tiny incisions to introduce a camera and small instruments, open surgery needs a bigger incision for direct access to the cyst and its removal.

When Open Procedures Are Preferable To Arthroscopic

In general, open surgery is selected under the following circumstances:

Size and Location: Open surgery may be necessary to provide a larger exposure for ganglion cysts that are large or deeply buried within joints or tissues.

Complexity: Open surgery enables greater visualization and careful dissection if the cyst is related to deeper structures or if there are concerns about surrounding nerves or blood arteries.

Failed Previous Procedures: Open surgery may be required to guarantee total eradication if conservative or arthroscopic therapies have proven futile or if the cyst has returned after previous care.

Patient Factors: The decision to proceed with open surgery may be influenced by a patient's anatomy, medical history, or the type of cyst they have.

Method By Step For Removing Open Cysts

Preparation: Depending on the location and complexity of the cyst, the patient is either put under general or regional anesthesia to undergo surgery.

Incision: Usually made right over the cyst, the incision site is marked with a surgical marker. The size and location of the cyst determine how big the incision should be.

Exposure: The cyst and its surrounding components are made visible when the surgeon makes an incision and carefully slices through the layers of skin, fat, and maybe muscle.

Identification of the Cyst: The cyst is located and isolated from the surrounding tissues using surgical tools and methods.

 If the cyst is connected to a tendon or joint capsule, careful dissection is necessary to guarantee total excision.

Closure: The surgical site is carefully examined to make sure no cyst remnants are left behind after the cyst and any related tissue have been removed.

Following the application of a sterile dressing, the incision is sealed with staples or sutures.

Possible Dangers And Issues

Although ganglion cyst removal with open surgery is generally safe, there are several dangers and possible side effects to be aware of:

Infection: The potential of infection at the site of incision or in deeper tissues exists with any surgical treatment.

Nerve or Vascular Injury: With cautious surgical skill, damage to adjacent nerves or blood arteries during dissection is unlikely, although it is conceivable.

Scar Formation: Compared to smaller incisions utilized in arthroscopic operations, the size of the incision may have a greater impact on scar formation.

Pain or Stiffness: Following surgery, some patients may have brief pain or stiffness in the afflicted joint or area; this normally goes away with rehabilitation.

Long-Term Results And Experiences Of Patients

Following open surgical excision of ganglion cysts, patients frequently report dramatic improvement in symptoms including pain, discomfort, and limited mobility brought on by the cyst.

If the cyst is fully removed, long-term results are usually good and the recurrence rate is minimal.

The size, location, and healing process of the individual can all affect how long it takes to recover from a cyst.

It could be suggested to do physical therapy or rehabilitation activities to fully recover the damaged joint or area's range of motion.

Follow-up consultations provide the surgeon with the chance to assess any potential issues and track the healing process.

All things considered, open surgery is still a good course of treatment for ganglion cyst removal when complete removal and the best possible results are of the utmost importance, even though it requires a longer process than arthroscopy.

CHAPTER SIX

RESTORATION AS WELL AS RECOVERY

Physical Therapy's Significance After Surgery

One of the most important aspects of the recovery process after ganglion cyst excision is physical therapy.

Due to the healing process and the production of scar tissue, it is typical for the affected joint or area to have stiffness and limited mobility following surgery.

Physical therapy uses focused exercises and strategies to restore function, strength, and range of motion to treat these problems.

A professional physical therapist will tailor a rehabilitation plan to the patient's unique requirements and the site of the cyst ectomy.

At the beginning of treatment, passive stretching and mild motions may be the major strategies used to keep joints flexible and avoid stiffness.

The therapist will progressively add more vigorous exercises to strengthen the surrounding muscles and enhance overall joint stability as the patient heals.

Ensuring the patient can achieve complete functional ability in the damaged area is one of the main objectives of physical therapy after surgery.

Exercises that imitate everyday tasks or, if appropriate, motions particular to a sport could be included in this.

Patients can regain confidence in their ability to use the injured joint without worrying about discomfort or re-injury by progressively reintroducing these motions under the supervision of a therapist.

Physical therapy also reduces the possibility of post-surgical problems such as muscle atrophy, joint stiffness, and aberrant movement patterns.

To maximize healing and improve recovery outcomes, the therapist may employ modalities such as manual methods, heat or ice therapy, and therapeutic exercises.

Following the recommended physical therapy routine is essential to long-term success and reducing the likelihood of recurrence or related problems.

Exercises For Strengthening And Restoring Joints

Targeted workouts are crucial to progressively restoring joint strength and mobility after ganglion cyst excision.

The location of the cyst and the damaged joint, as well as the person's general health and fitness level, will determine the precise activities that are advised.

Gentle range-of-motion exercises are frequently the main emphasis of the first post-surgery exercises to prevent stiffness and increase circulation in the affected area.

These could involve aided or passive motions carried out with the help of a physical therapist. The focus switches to active range-of-motion exercises that the patient may do on their own as recovery advances and pain decreases.

A physical therapist may recommend resistance exercises employing body weight, free weights, or resistance bands to strengthen the muscles surrounding the injured joint. As the patient's strength increases, the intensity of these workouts is meant to be gradually increased.

Exercises that build strength assist in stabilizing the joint, promote healing, and fend off further damage or problems.

To enhance joint stability and coordination, the rehabilitation program may also incorporate balance and proprioception exercises.

Patients who engage in activities requiring precise movement patterns or weight-bearing on the afflicted joint should pay special attention to these exercises.

The physical therapist closely evaluates the patient's development during the rehabilitation process and modifies the training regimen as necessary. To keep the program safe and successful, patients must report any pain or difficulties they have during activities.

CHAPTER SEVEN

A COMMON QUESTION AND A FAQ

Will The Cyst Return Once It Has Been Removed?

When thinking about having a ganglion cyst removed, one common worry is that the cyst might come back. It's critical to realize that, even while surgical excision usually attempts to remove the cyst entirely, recurrence is a remote possibility.

This may happen if the surgery fails to remove the complete cyst wall or if the cyst reappears as a result of joint stress or damage.

Surgeons usually try to remove the visible cyst together with the surrounding tissue and joint capsule to decrease the chance of regrowth and lessen the risk of recurrence.

Furthermore, adhering strictly to post-operative care instructions—such as immobilizing the injured joint and performing recommended rehabilitation exercises—can help promote a full recovery and lower the risk of recurrence.

Scheduling routine follow-up visits with your physician is also essential. These checkups enable early detection of any recurrence signals and enable timely intervention if necessary.

All in all, a satisfactory outcome is promoted by comprehensive surgical removal and careful aftercare, which considerably reduce the possibility of recurrence.

How Much Time Does Recovery Following Surgery Take?

The length of recovery following ganglion cyst excision surgery varies from patient to patient and is influenced by variables such as the cyst's location and size, the patient's ability to heal, and compliance with post-operative care guidelines. After the operation, most patients may usually return to their regular activities in a few weeks.

To lessen swelling and accelerate recovery, patients are usually instructed to rest and elevate the injured limb right after surgery. Painkillers could be recommended to ease discomfort in the early stages after recovery. It could be suggested to have an outpatient procedure or a brief hospital stay, depending on the intricacy of the surgery and the patient's general condition.

Exercises for physical therapy or rehabilitation may also be recommended to help the afflicted joint regain strength and mobility. It's critical to adhere to the rehabilitation regimen prescribed by your physician to maximize healing and avoid complications.

It is common to have some edema, bruising, stiffness, or mild discomfort in the area surrounding the surgery site throughout the recuperation phase. Usually, these symptoms get better over time. To prevent strain or harm to the healing tissues, patients are recommended to refrain from heavy lifting or vigorous activities until cleared by their healthcare physician.

With careful adherence to post-operative instructions, regular follow-up sessions, and sufficient healing time, the majority of patients can anticipate a full recovery following ganglion cyst excision surgery.

Are Ganglion Cysts Avoidable?

Since the precise etiology of ganglion cysts isn't always known, preventing them completely is difficult. Nonetheless, there are a few tactics that can lessen the chance of getting these cysts or having a recurrence following therapy.

Avoiding recurrent joint stress or damage is one strategy to prevent ganglion cyst formation. This includes employing protective gear and following appropriate ergonomics when engaging in joint-stressing activities like manual labor or sports.

Stretching and regular exercise can also help to maintain healthy joint health. Enhancing the strength of the muscles surrounding the joints can improve stability and support while possibly lowering the likelihood of cyst formation.

Speak with a healthcare professional about preventive actions specific to your situation if you have a history of ganglion cysts or are predisposed to joint-related problems. They can offer tailored advice to reduce your risk of getting ganglion cysts depending on your lifestyle and medical history.

Adopting these preventative steps will help maintain general joint health and may eventually lower the likelihood of ganglion cyst formation, even if total prevention may not always be possible.

Do any alternatives to surgery for treatment?

If a ganglion cyst is bothersome or interferes with everyday activities, surgery is usually advised.

Alternative therapies, however, might occasionally be taken into consideration, particularly for tiny or asymptomatic cysts.

Aspiration is a non-surgical procedure in which a medical professional uses a needle to remove fluid from a cyst. This treatment can be carried out in an office or clinic under local anesthetic. Compared to surgical removal, aspiration is less intrusive and typically results in a speedier recovery period; nonetheless, there is an increased risk of cyst recurrence.

Injections of corticosteroids are an additional alternate treatment. Corticosteroids injected directly into the cyst may help lower inflammation and briefly relieve symptoms. Patients who choose not to have surgery or those with cysts that are extremely challenging to approach surgically may find this option appropriate.

It's crucial to remember that although these non-traditional therapies may relieve symptoms, they cannot remove the cyst or stop it from returning in the future. The size, location, symptoms, and personal preferences of each patient all play a role in the decision between surgery and non-surgical treatments. Speaking with a healthcare professional can assist in figuring out the best course of action for your particular situation.

What Dangers Come With Not Getting A Ganglion Cyst Treated?

Even though ganglion cysts are usually benign and painless, delaying treatment can eventually result in problems and discomfort. Untreated ganglion cysts run the risk of growing larger and putting pressure on nearby blood arteries, nerves, or tissues. The affected area may become painful, numb, tingly, or weak as a result of this pressure.

Untreated ganglion cysts can occasionally impair joint function and movement, particularly if they form close to a joint or tendon. This may restrict movement and increase the difficulty or discomfort of daily tasks.

The possibility of a cyst rupturing or fluid leaking into the surrounding tissues is another risk. Inflammation, pain, and an elevated risk of infection might result from a ruptured cyst in the affected area. Antibiotics or extra medical intervention may be necessary in cases of infection, which can further complicate treatment.

Untreated ganglion cysts can also worry some people about their looks, particularly if the cyst is noticeable or large. This may affect one's quality of life and sense of self, especially if the cyst is visible, as on the hand or wrist.

In summary, although prompt treatment for ganglion cysts may not always be necessary, it is crucial to regularly monitor these lesions and consult a physician if symptoms arise to avoid potential problems and maintain optimal joint health and function.

www.ingramcontent.com/pod-product-compliance
Lightning Source LLC
Chambersburg PA
CBHW071216260726
48653CB00041B/873